MAGN

What Your Doctor Needs You to Know

Nolan Edwards

Including: How to Fight Diabetes, Have a Healthy Heart, and Get Strong Bones!

Disclaimer

Before implementing advisement from this informative, consult your physician first to be sure it is appropriate for you. If you are unsure of any foods recommended, you should always consult your physician's advice. Remember to talk with your doctor about the potential drug interactions and correct dosage before taking any magnesium supplements. The information in this book reflects the author's opinions and is not intended to replace medical advice.

The author has made every effort to supply accurate information in the creation of this book. The author offers no warranty and accepts no responsibility for any loss or damages of any kind that may be incurred by the reader as a result of actions arising from the use of the contents in this book. The reader assumes all responsibility for the use of the information in this text.

Table of Contents

Chapter 1: Introduction

Has your doctor ever told you that magnesium is the most important nutrient for your health?

If not, then you have overlooked the chance to alleviate many of your current, as well as prevent future, bodily disorders. Magnesium helps to maintain nerve function, supports a healthy immune system, keeps bones strong, and performs normal heart pumping. While actively used in over 300 biochemical reactions, magnesium: helps to promote normal blood pressure, is involved in protein synthesis, speeds up the body's metabolism, and regulates blood sugar levels. There is an increased interest in the role of magnesium in managing and preventing disorders such as cardiovascular disease, hypertension, and diabetes.

Magnesium's uses are plenty. One use is alleviating constipation through certain forms of the mineral. If you have ever bought laxative medicines in the past, flip the cover and read the active ingredients. You will find that it includes one of these forms.

Magnesium is also a calcium channel blocker. This means that it aids calcium in lowering blood pressure. It is possible that you already know the importance of calcium for your bones, but those bones become what is termed 'healthy bones' only with the help of magnesium. The most concerning part is that people tend to take calcium pills without realizing that magnesium is not present for proper absorption. So overall, you may need more magnesium than calcium, especially for people with osteoporosis.

What about your energy powerhouse? Yes, I mean your heart. Magnesium protects the heart and helps the heart muscle function better. Strokes and heart attacks can be prevented by magnesium as it is a natural blood thinner, much like Aspirin. It helps to protect your blood vessels—where most cardiovascular diseases take place.

Magnesium helps to prevent diabetes. There is a correlation between diabetes and magnesium levels. People with normal or higher levels of magnesium do not typically have diabetes; those with lower than normal levels are more prone to diabetes.

Magnesium is present in soil. Certified organic foods and those from local Farmers Markets have substantially higher quantities of magnesium than conventional farms. Soil from commercial farmlands are deplete of magnesium due to a lack of crop rotation as well as land rest. They habitually replenish the soil with nitrogen, phosphorus, and potassium, leaving out magnesium.

Magnesium nourishes the production and quality of crops grown in the earth. It is also necessary for the well-being of animals and people consuming these plants. Along with other minerals, magnesium has to be present in the soil where food is grown.

All in all, you will discover more about how magnesium affects your blood, glucose, energy, hormones, muscles, nerves, bones, and some of the most common disorders associated with a lack of it.

Indispensable to your health and well-being, magnesium continues to be an essential nutrient. This book is about the importance of magnesium and the crucial role it plays throughout the human body. Knowing magnesium's linkage to each of your body systems and functions will better allow you to alleviate and guard against long-term threats, disorders, and ailments.

Over the past 100 years, the dietary intake of magnesium has gone down dramatically. Between 67% to 82% of Americans are magnesium deficient. The incidence of bodily disorders is lower in people when magnesium levels are higher. More than eight million deaths occurred due to sudden cardiac failure in the United States between the years 1941 and 1995 on account of magnesium deficiency. Known by medical researchers and scientists for years, magnesium is the most common and vital mineral that can help alleviate diseases and problems for a longer and healthier life. In proper dosage, this mineral does not have any registered side effects.

Many drugs are designed to relieve the symptoms of heart disease, though the cause is not eliminated. In this guide, you will discover a step-by-step process as to how a natural mineral can help you regain your health and improve body functioning. Balanced hormones, a healthy cardiovascular system, well-functioning detoxification pathways, healthy nervous system, strong teeth, and bones all depend on the magnesium sufficiency.

Daily Intake

Recommended daily allowance by the Current U.S policy of magnesium for adults aged 30+ is:

- 320 mg per day for women
- 360 mg per day for pregnant women
- 420 mg per day for men

According to some medical experts, the said amounts of magnesium are insufficient for people who are suffering from health problems. For example, nutritionist and doctors recommended 500mg or more of magnesium for people suffering from low blood pressure, menstrual cramping, glucose depletion and other common disorders. To meet their bodily needs, certain individuals and those with particular problems are more prone to deficiency and may require additional supplements and intake of magnesium. Such individuals and such problems may include drug or alcohol consumption, diabetes, certain medications like cancer-fighting drug Cisplatin and Diuretics.

Present throughout the full landscape of human physiology, magnesium is the basic building block of life. It is known to be present in an ionic form which means that it supplies the body with the type of minerals that it promptly recognizes and quickly absorbs.

Forms of Magnesium Intake

Magnesium is known in many forms, but typically is used as a supplement. They can vary by delivery and type. Some of them include: Magnesium Hydroxide, Magnesium Sulfate, Magnesium Bicarbonate, Magnesium Oxide, Magnesium Chloride, and Magnesium Phosphate.

A new form of magnesium supplementation is transdermal magnesium, which is affordable, accessible, and convenient. Also known as 'topical', it is particularly helpful for increasing magnesium intake when oral supplements are not working. It is a fantastic choice for people suffering from diarrhea, low tolerance for oral magnesium, or other intestinal problems. Examples of transdermal forms of magnesium include Epsom salts, magnesium oil, and magnesium salts. Magnesium oil is the most potent form of transdermal supplementing.

Chapter 2: Magnesium and Your Blood

It is important for all of us above 30 years old to be cognoscente of our blood pressure. This is because the risk of high blood pressure is increased with age.

According to new findings, magnesium plays an important role in people suffering from high blood pressure by reducing it. Results from epidemiological studies have revealed that people with more potassium, calcium, and magnesium in their bodies have a reduced risk of hypertension (high blood pressure).

In 1992, a randomized trial was conducted in which researchers recruited 150 people to take part in the placebo-controlled, double- blinded test. The assigned subjects included a placebo or a daily supplement of magnesium oxide for 12 weeks.

At first, no significant differences were observed, but later there was a significant decrease in both diastolic blood pressure (the pressure in your arteries when the heart rests between beats) and systolic blood pressure (When your heart pumps it pushes and contracts blood through the arteries to the rest of your body. The force created puts pressure on the arteries. This pressure is known as systolic blood pressure) in the magnesium group.

One out of every three persons has hypertension or high blood pressure. Hypertension is very problematic because it can damage your body quietly without giving a hint of its work. You may develop the symptoms later on, but until then the damage might be done. Uncontrolled hypertension is said to be a serious and common health concern that can increase the risk of strokes and heart problems. Symptoms or warning signs are not often known. A few symptoms are a poor quality of life, disabilities, and heart attacks. These magnesium deficient health risks are what your doctor wants you to be aware of.

If your blood pressure is between 125/80 and 135/80 then you are diagnosed with pre-hypertension. Giving your body its required amount of magnesium is a good start toward reducing your blood pressure through lifestyle modifications. How? Read on...

What Causes High Blood Pressure?

High blood pressure is inversely connected to magnesium deficiency. As one goes up, the other goes down. If you are magnesium deficient, your body produces too much insulin. Your blood pressure increases as your insulin level rises.

The effects of high blood pressure are wide ranging. The debilitating effects of high insulin, leptin, and blood glucose levels give proof of the linkage between hypertension (abnormally high blood pressure) and insulin resistance. If you are struggling with high blood pressure, then it is highly recommended that you get your magnesium levels tested.

How Magnesium Promotes Healthy Blood Pressure and Heart Function

For the stabilization of blood pressure, magnesium and calcium provide an essential connection. If magnesium is your go-to supplement, then you will want the complementary mineral, calcium.

Most calcium and magnesium supplements contain a ratio of one part magnesium to two parts calcium. "The logic behind this ratio is based on the relative amounts of these nutrients used in the body. But in order to determine how much we might need to take as a supplement, we should consider how much of the nutrients are recycled and stored in our body and how much nutrients we are getting in our food."[1]

So in short, you should have both. Magnesium assists your body in absorbing and retaining calcium.

Typically you would be consuming twice as much magnesium as calcium. This ratio is consistent and beneficial for most. There are certain individuals who can benefit from a different proportion, however. People with kidney and heart diseases require different ratios. Too much magnesium can aggravate these pre-existing symptoms, so a balance between both is necessary.

Since the 1930's, magnesium has been prescribed as the remedial cure for heart disease. Seven major clinical studies observed a reduction in the odds of death by more than 50% of patients suffering from heart disease. One of the studies showed that magnesium must be given to the patient prior to taking any medicine, after the onset of a heart attack. The resultant studies showed that if followed correctly, hypertension, heart muscle damage, and arrhythmia are significantly reduced.

How Does Magnesium Benefit Your Heart Exactly?

Responsible for the heart muscle functioning; in the same way that, "it helps nerve functions throughout the body, magnesium is essential for coordinating the activity of the heart muscle and the nerves that initiate the heartbeat. If your magnesium levels are low, you are more likely to be at risk for arrhythmias (irregular heartbeats) and heart palpitations."[2]

Magnesium aids the heart by:

1. Dilating the constricted blood vessels

2. Reducing heart muscle damage and hypertension

3. Dissolving blood clots

4. Acting as an antioxidant that prevents free radicals from forming at the site of an injury

5. Preventing spasms in the blood vessel walls and heart muscle

6. Preventing arrhythmia and dramatically lessening the site of injury

7. Counteracting an imbalance of calcium which can induce spasms

Do We Have Enough Magnesium?

In today's world, more than 80% of the people have a deficiency in magnesium.

The problem is that low magnesium levels cannot be diagnosed by symptoms alone. Low lab tests cannot give accurate readings of the amount of Magnesium in your tissues. A sample of magnesium can be taken by distributing one percent of the magnesium in your body to your blood. This method is not accurate enough to diagnose anyone. Therefore, relying too much on blood tests for magnesium evidence, and not on signs and symptoms of magnesium deficiency, can equate to a misdiagnosis.

Signs and Symptoms

Some signs and symptoms of magnesium deficiency include:

Spasms or muscle soreness
Irritability
Headaches
Inability to sleep or insomnia
High level of stress
Sensitivity to noise
Difficulty in concentrating or fuzzy brain
Thyroid
Kidney stones
Gut Disorder
Constipation
Lack of appetite

If you have more than five of the above symptoms, then you may greatly benefit from magnesium supplementation. The other option (instead of supplementation) is to consume it through organically bound elements.

Lower your Blood Pressure Naturally

Here are some smart strategies to lower your blood pressure naturally:

1. Optimizing your Vitamin D levels: normalizing your vitamin D levels has a powerful effect on stabilizing your blood sugar.

2. Exercise: Consisting of aerobics, strength, and core training, an effective exercise program, sprinting or burst-type exercises can help lower your blood sugar levels thus normalizing your blood pressure.

3. Use of stress management techniques: Your blood pressure can increase alarmingly by mild stress.

4. Eating: Foods such as sugar type grains and other food may raise your insulin. Therefore, they should be avoided if you have high blood pressure. These foods include cereal, pasta, potatoes, breads and rice. Your nutritional diet should contain healthy foods and less insulin boosting foods. Particularly helpful is crushed raw garlic.

None of the above tips include a blood pressure drug, so the criteria for 'natural' remains. Taking natural remedies is advantageous because too many blood pressure drugs can cause diseases like type 2 diabetes, diarrhea, and cancer. However, if your blood levels are unusually high, then you do need to go on medication. Otherwise, you may have a stroke or permanent brain damage, both of which are irreversible.

If you follow the prescribed tips and magnesium related points from above then your levels may soon lower, and you can hopefully begin slow down your medications. Adding magnesium is important in making progress in your health.

Chapter 3: Magnesium and Insulin

We will review how magnesium is the foundation and structure of life. So as we follow magnesium and its benefits, we will begin to understand what role it plays in our life. The intent of this chapter is to understand magnesium, its meaning towards medicinal health and how glucose plays an important role in it.

Insulin is the hormone directly tied to the increasing cause of high sugar levels. It is secreted by the pancreas, where a group of cells called the islet cells carries out the secretion. Insulin has many functions that are more important than we realize. If properly combined in a balanced way with magnesium, insulin can help in regulating:

1. Blood sugar
2. Magnesium levels in our body
3. Growth hormones
4. Retention of sodium levels
5. Liver functions
6. Blood lipids
7. Cholesterol in the body
8. Stores of protein
9. Cell division

10. Fat in the body
11. Muscle Building
12. Testosterone, estrogen, and progesterone

Present throughout the full landscape of human physiology, magnesium is the basic building block of life. It is known to be present in an ionic form which means that it supplies the body with the type of minerals that it promptly recognizes and quickly absorbs.

Magnesium is both necessary for the manufacturing of insulin as well as the action of insulin. One role of blood cells is to transport magnesium throughout the body and for this, insulin is required.

A recent study conducted by Dr. Jerry Nadler of the Gonda Diabetes Center at the City of Hope Medical Center in California found that 16 healthy persons, when placed on magnesium-deficient diets, had higher chances of having both heart disease and diabetes. Their insulin became less effective at getting sugar from their blood into their fuel cells than those who were not on magnesium-deficient diets. [4]

Magnesium plays a primary function in preventing insulin deregulation (Abnormalities of insulin metabolism) and type 2 diabetes.

Hyperglycemia

Hyperglycemia, also commonly known as type 2 diabetes, is the most prevalent form of diabetes. In this condition, the blood sugar levels increase faster than the other types of diabetes. Your body is not able to take advantage of this potential energy or use the insulin produced.

Magnesium Wasting Disease

Magnesium wasting disease is a disorder that can result in disturbances in nearly every organ and can cause potentially fatal complications.

This disease often occurs when insulin processing becomes problematic, and magnesium gets excreted out of the body through the urine. Magnesium wasting disease is mainly caused by an improper functioning of the pancreas. Since the pancreas is unable to function properly, it causes a decrease in insulin secretion. If insulin levels are low, magnesium is not transported to the body cells. This disruption is a common disorder in diabetic patients, as well.

Problems associated with insulin resistance decreases insulin secretion and impair glucose tolerance including intracellular magnesium (production of magnesium) and low serum (levels of potassium.) Insulin resistance is a state in which the pancreas resists the reproduction of insulin. This is primarily due to improper pancreatic function. Impaired glucose tolerance is a pre-diabetic state of hyperglycemia (a condition in which excess amount of glucose circulates the body). Increased risk of type 2 diabetes occurs from lower serum and dietary magnesium. Sometimes, redistribution of magnesium takes place in the cells by insulin. Magnesium is delivered to the same cell twice or more, which leads to an excessive amount, which causes 'low serum magnesium'.

Your cells need to store your body's daily required amount of magnesium; otherwise an increase in blood pressure is observed. Remember, this is because insulin is not able to transport magnesium into the body cells. Reduction in magnesium also makes our blood vessels constrict.

Insulin and Cholesterol

Insulin is said to regulate cholesterol levels; restricted insulin will not be able to do so, which later on contributes to higher cholesterol levels and causes cardiovascular disease, osteoporosis, and metabolic complications.

The cholesterol magnesium story points out "that magnesium is another useful nutrient for treating raised cholesterol."[5] In one study, magnesium at a dose of 430mg per day was shown to reduce cholesterol levels.

Insulin Resistance and Insulin Sensitivity

"Insulin sensitivity describes how sensitive the body is to the effects of insulin. Someone said to be insulin sensitive will require smaller amounts of insulin to lower blood glucose levels than someone who has low sensitivity." [6]

Insulin resistance is a condition where, once your insulin levels decrease, the pancreas produces extra insulin to compensate for the loss. However, later on, the pancreas is not able to make a continuous surplus of insulin to keep your sugar levels at bay. This results in type 2 diabetes.

A resistance to the 'hormone insulin' results in an increasing 'blood sugar insulin resistance'. However, upping your intake of magnesium will reduce this problem by improving insulin sensitivity. Insulin sensitivity is a good thing! The pancreas detects the decrease in insulin levels. This detection period is known as insulin sensitivity. The faster the detection, the better the insulin sensitivity. Insulin sensitivity improvement means improving the function of the insulin-producing organ, the pancreas.

Insulin and magnesium need each other. Without insulin, the secretion from the pancreas will not be able to control your blood sugar levels. In other words, it will not be efficient. Without magnesium, your pancreas cannot secrete enough insulin.

An increase in magnesium intake will adjust sensitivity to insulin by the pancreas. The pancreas can detect lowering sugar levels that can improve metabolic syndrome, heart disease, menstrual cramping pre-diabetes and even diabetes. This reaction (that allows any drop in sugar detection) uses an intracellular enzyme called tyrosine kinase. As you can probably guess, this enzyme also requires magnesium.

People who take daily oral magnesium supplementation overall showed to have a 37% reduction in blood sugar and a 10% improvement in sensitivity. Abnormal lipoprotein patterns can also be corrected by magnesium. Doctors advise their patients to supplement magnesium in a correct way, meaning that oral methods and transdermal are combined using magnesium oil (liquid magnesium chloride).

Hypersecretion of Insulin

Hypersecretion of insulin and adrenalin compensate when magnesium levels fall. The constancy of the levels of intracellular magnesium in the soft tissues is maintained by increased secretion. Insulin tightly regulates the intracellular magnesium and plasma concentrations. When insulin modulates, a shift of magnesium from extracellular to intracellular space occurs.

Plague build-up was noticed when insulin floats in the blood. This is because insulin causes endothelial proliferation. In every step, insulin increases the chances of causing cardiovascular disease. It constricts the arteries, fills the body with excess sugar and stimulates the sympathetic nervous system. It also, increases platelet adhesiveness of the blood.

Chapter 4: Magnesium and Your Energy

Low on energy? A commonly overlooked mineral for energy, magnesium can supercharge you throughout your day.

Out of the many biochemical reactions magnesium performs, producing energy out of glucose is one of them. So when your glucose levels are low, your energy can drop.

A recent study done by the Department of Agriculture Human Nutrition Research Center in Grand Forks, N.D, revealed that women who had higher heart rates and required more oxygen to do physical tasks were magnesium deficient. Later on, when their magnesium levels were restored, they were able to complete tasks more efficiently. The harder your body works (without magnesium), the more depleted you will feel. [7]

How Magnesium Helps Your Energy Levels

Magnesium aids in the making of the primary form of energy- ATP (adenosine triphosphate). Therefore, a deficiency in magnesium can make you tired or low in energy.

For maintaining proper magnesium levels, consumption of supplements may not be a good idea. Throughout the day, your body needs a steady supply of magnesium. Due to bulk, most supplements will not contain more than 110 mg of magnesium. The easiest way to maintain your energy is to have a rich diet of magnesium.

Your body consistently uses up your storage of magnesium that you had after breakfast. Eating a magnesium diet throughout the day is quite sufficient instead of taking it all at once. This will help in keeping the magnesium levels elevated.

How Do You Promote Magnesium Absorption?

The absorption of magnesium in the gut can be attained by consuming vitamin B, especially vitamin B6.

Vitamin B12 is also a vitamin that helps keep the body's nerve and blood cells able while strengthening DNA, the genetic material in all cells. Vitamin B12 helps prevent a type of anemia called megaloblastic anemia that makes people tired and weak. So if you are not tired or weak, the absorption power of your body is highly increased. This means that more magnesium will be absorbed by your body, if your energy is high.

Stop Draining Your Body of Magnesium!

Yes, you are indirectly responsible for the decrease in your energy levels, due to a decrease in magnesium. Though you are not fully aware, excessive coffee, alcohol, sodas, sugar, and salt can reduce your magnesium levels—causing energy drop.

Magnesium carbonate, gluconate, sulfate, and oxide should be avoided; these are the most poorly absorbed forms. In this case, you would deprive your body of magnesium because you think you are already taking your daily dosage.

On the opposite side of the spectrum, too much magnesium can inadvertently drain your body of the mineral. Notice that too much magnesium can cause side effects which includes diarrhea because it promotes bowel motility. "Magnesium is often balanced with calcium because 'calcium constipates and magnesium moves' when it comes to bowel activity." [8]

Magnesium attracts and retains fluid in the bowels. Magnesium also relaxes muscle spasms and increases cellular energy production to energize the colon.

Most bowel activity can be avoided by switching to magnesium glycinate (the gentlest form on the stomach). Magnesium glycinate is the best-absorbed form of magnesium, so taking a lower dosage of this is preferred over taking higher doses in other forms. Most importantly, taking magnesium glycinate does not cause gastrointestinal distress or loose stools as with other forms of magnesium. Please see the end chapter on forms for further information.

Chapter 5: Magnesium and Hormones

Are you struggling with pregnancy issues? Are you excessively hungry or tired? Does your mood sink like the Titanic before your periods? The most probable reason could be that you are deficient in magnesium. For almost all hormonal conditions, magnesium is prescribed as the first antidote. It is especially effective for:

PCOS (Polycystic Ovary Syndrome): A hormonal disorder that causes enlargening of the ovaries accompanied by tiny cysts on the outer edges.

Hair loss: Dandruff, scalp burn, and hair fall.

Thyroid: Any dysfunction of the butterfly-shaped gland at the base of the neck.

Menopause: A naturally occurring decline in reproductive hormones during a woman's midlife - between ages 40 and 55.

Adrenal Fatigue: It is a term related to non-specific symptoms such as sleep disturbances, fatigue, digestive problems, body aches and nervousness.

PMS: A group of pre menstruation symptoms that occur in women, typically between ovulation and a period.

The positive fact about magnesium is that the effects are immediate.

Why Are We So Deficient in Magnesium? What's Wrong with This Mineral?

The reason for our major lack in this mineral is that during stress our cells dump magnesium. To cope with daily life, we actively decrease the mineral density in our bodies as a way to boost our nervous system.

A sluggish day can be revved up by a properly working nervous system. If you commute, work tirelessly, worry or drink coffee, then you may want to question if you are deficient in your magnesium levels.

How Magnesium Can Affect...

PMS: Your cravings for magnesium-rich foods (like chocolate) increases before your period. Ever wondered why? Your body requires more magnesium due to its decline. During a woman's cycle, magnesium levels tend to fluctuate. Your magnesium levels decrease with the increase in progesterone or estrogen levels. Magnesium plummets when both progesterone and estrogen are elevated during the second half of the menstrual cycle. This causes spasms in the brain arteries- a prelude to migraines and PMS. PMS- related symptoms, such as headaches, dizziness, sugar cravings, migraines, low blood sugar, and fluid retention can be relieved by increasing supplemental and dietary magnesium.

Tips to Deal with…

Dysmenorrhea (painful periods): Consider taking magnesium before your periods arrive. Women can get relief from painful periods by taking high doses of magnesium. Doses should start with 350 mg of powdered magnesium citrate and can be increased to 1000 mg to 1,250 mg, if needed. (Again, consult your doctor)

Infertility: If you are having trouble becoming pregnant, low magnesium is a probable culprit. Egg implantation will more likely be prevented if you are magnesium deficient. Magnesium deficiency causes spasms in a woman's fallopian tube, which in turn affects the eggs.

Pregnancy: At least 370mg of magnesium is a must for pregnant women. Daily consumption of magnesium throughout pregnancy can reduce the risk of premature births, sudden infant death syndrome, pre-eclampsia, and other complications.

Weight: Enzymes that control absorption, digestion, and the use of proteins, carbohydrates, and fats are activated by increasing magnesium levels. Energy is formed in the body when insulin is enabled to escort glucose into the cells as needed. If there is not enough magnesium in the body, both glucose and insulin levels become elevated. When insulin does not function properly, excessive glucose is stored in the body as fat—mostly around your middle section. Chronic magnesium deficiency can lead to anxiety, obesity, diabetes, and hypoglycemia (post diabetic period).

Eight Ways Magnesium Can Rescue Your Hormones

1. **Magnesium regulates cortisol**: Magnesium prevents excessive cortisol (symptoms are skin irritation, allergic reactions, and other types of skin problems) and calms your nervous system. Your central hormonal system, called the hypothalamic pituitary adrenal axis or HPA, deals with your stress hormonal system that gets aggravated due to high cortisol levels. Hormones function better when cortisol is regulated, including your sex and thyroid hormones.

2. **Magnesium lowers your blood sugar**: As explained in the second chapter, magnesium plays an important role in bringing down your blood sugar levels. Magnesium is very effective in sensitizing insulin receptors. These play an indispensable part in the regulation of glucose homeostasis. This functional process, under degenerate conditions, may manifest in a range of clinical phenomenon including diabetes and cancer. Better insulin control results in fewer sugar cravings. Healthy insulin sensitivity is important for osteoporosis and weight loss, and it also helps prevent PCOS.

3. **Magnesium and thyroid**: For the production of thyroid hormones, magnesium is essential. It is anti-inflammatory (reduces inflammation or swelling) which helps to treat cases of thyroid disease and aids the autoimmune inflammation (swelling). Other ways you can address thyroid autoimmunity include selenium supplement and gluten elimination (reduction of fatty foods).

4. **Magnesium aids sleep**: Magnesium plays an important role in our sleeping patterns, but too much or too less can cause sleep disturbances. Overall, magnesium is a great sleep-promoter. It is also great for hormone production sleep is very crucial. Sleep is when we should have a surge in anabolic hormones like growth hormone and DHEA. Proper magnesium ratios are vitally important in order to correctly use calcium in the cells. A calcium imbalance causes cell death and calcification; that in turn is caused by a deficiency in magnesium. This can tie into the brain and its secretions through the pituitary gland for aiding in the circadian rhythm; further leading to symptoms like menstrual cramping, heart trouble, and muscle cramps.

5. **Magnesium makes hormones**: Magnesium is involved in the manufacturing of steroid hormones such as testosterone, progesterone, and estrogen. In direct relation, magnesium has also been shown to reduce hot flashes by 50 percent.

6. **Magnesium activates vitamin D**: Responsible for enhancing intestinal absorption of calcium, iron, magnesium, phosphate, and zinc; vitamin D cannot do its jobs without magnesium. Too much vitamin D supplementation and not enough of the pure form can cause magnesium deficiency. You also need to consume it in your food as well as take supplemental vitamin K2 with more magnesium. "Taking mega doses of vitamin D supplements without sufficient amounts of K2 and magnesium can lead to vitamin D toxicity and magnesium deficiency symptoms, which include inappropriate calcification." [9]

7. **Magnesium is used to fuel cellular energy**: Magnesium is so intricately involved with Krebs cycle (ATP energy production) and glycolysis that we can safely say that without magnesium there is no cellular energy. Glandular tissue like testes, thyroid, and ovaries is metabolically very active, and thus it requires more magnesium and cellular energy than any other tissue.

8. **Magnesium is anti-aging**: The mineral has been shown to enhance the production of glutathione, prevent telomere shortening, and reduce oxidative stress.

Chapter 6: Magnesium and Muscles

Magnesium is a powerful element for treating muscle pain as well as building them. There are many people who are completely unaware of all the benefits magnesium holds for helping relieve pain as well as boost muscles.

Muscles and nerves rely on magnesium for their functions. Not receiving enough magnesium debilitates this duo from cycling properly. Problems in muscle contraction and relaxation, aka cramping, occur as a result. Calcium absorption is necessary for muscles to contract, while magnesium is vital to their retraction. Keep in mind that since human bodies are not able to efficiently store magnesium, it is crucial to ensure that your diet is rich in it.

Magnesium and calcium work to help regulate the muscle tone and the body's nerves. Magnesium decides the amount of calcium to be allowed into nerve cells. The nerve activates if there is an uncontrolled rush of calcium into a nerve cell. This over-activation of the nerve causes disorders as this nerve sends too many messages to the muscles resulting in a muscle that gets cramped or over-contracted

Yes, this discussion is leading to chronic pain of the muscle variety. Not only will you have pain, but also muscle cramping and fatigue; all because your magnesium levels need a boost.

Magnesium is a Quick Remedy for Muscle Pain

Especially for muscle pain, you can apply magnesium cream, magnesium oil, or Epsom salt (which is rich in magnesium) directly onto the skin.

There are even more ways that magnesium can be better absorbed. Try taking a magnesium oil or Epsom salt foot bath. Let your feet soak in the magnesium oil/Epsom salt for about sixty minutes- this will allow enough time for letting your foot absorb all the magnesium it needs.

Muscle Functioning

According to the University of Maryland Medical Center, Magnesium plays a crucial role in the healthy function of your muscles. If you have spasms or muscle pain, then magnesium may help in relaxation of muscle tissues. It also blocks excessive calcium from depositing in your muscles tissues.

Effects and Disorders

Magnesium could help treat joint and muscle aches due to any medical condition like osteoporosis, fibromyalgia, and restless leg syndrome. It also helps to ease your muscle pain associated with PMS, PCOS, and menopause. Magnesium can also treat a condition involving painful menstrual cramping known as dysmenorrhea. It can also be used to counter joint pain caused by rheumatoid arthritis.

Causes of Cramps

Muscle strain, overuse of a muscle, sitting in a position for a prolonged period of time, or dehydration may result in muscle cramping. Many muscle cramps are harmless, but some can be caused by underlying medical condition such as:

1. **Mineral Depletion**--- Too little magnesium, calcium, or potassium contributes to leg cramps. Depletion of these minerals can also be due to diuretic medication often prescribed for high blood pressure.

2. **Nerve Compression**--- Lumbar Stenosis (compression of nerves in your spine) produces pain in your legs resulting in cramps. The longer you walk, the more you will have pain. You can improve the onset of your symptoms by walking in a slightly flexed position.

3. **Inadequate Magnesium in the Blood Supply**---Conditions in which your arteries narrow, such as arteriosclerosis of the extremities, do not allow blood to flow through your body. Symptoms include a cramp-like pain in your feet and legs while you are working out.

Athletics and Magnesium

There are many benefits that magnesium supplementation can give you in improving your recovery, performance, and athletic training. There are many athletes who are completely unaware of this vital mineral, and many who do not consume it, which leads to a lack of post-exercise muscle recovery, impaired performance, and reduced exercise capacity. Magnesium proved to increase physical performance.

Magnesium is vital for your body's physiological processes such as muscle contraction, keeping your cells healthy, increasing energy production, and relaxing muscles.

Studies revealed that female endurance athletes were able to run for a longer duration of time when on magnesium supplements. There was an increase in VO2 max (your body's ability to convert and utilize oxygen for a boost in fitness). Therefore, a reduction in magnesium can cause symptoms such as reduced vigor training and declining performance because our body tends to eat up magnesium when you workout. Moreover, if magnesium is not available in plenty, energy is low, and this might cause these symptoms.

Muscle Cramps and Magnesium

As mentioned, magnesium is necessary for normal muscular relaxation and contraction. With the addition of magnesium supplements, increased incidence of muscle cramps can be avoided. In a recent study, swimmers with magnesium supplementation in their diets were found to have an 86% reduction in muscle cramps. If muscle cramps are a problem for you, then you could add magnesium supplementation to your nutritional regime. [10]

Better Muscle Recovery and Magnesium

Magnesium assists in post-exercise muscle recovery as well as structural damage to muscle cells. Therefore, it is crucial for maintaining muscle health.

A study showed that 1,453 adult people showed better muscle function and integrity if higher serum (blood) magnesium levels were present. These included: ankle extension strength, grip strength, knee extension torque and lower leg muscle power. These results highlighted how magnesium plays an important role in muscle recovery and formation.

Research and clinical experience in nerve pain conditions such as pancreatic cancer have shown that magnesium can dramatically lessen the associated pain. Although it is clear that magnesium can decrease muscle pain (it relaxes the muscles), why it helps with nerve pain was less clear.[11]

Chapter 7: Magnesium and Nerves

"Think of all the jobs the nervous system must perform. Every activity of life, from the respiration of a single cell to a gross motor function such as piloting an aircraft, is controlled by the nerves."[12]

To maintain a healthy nervous system, a number of chief nutrients occupy a role, including (you guessed it!), magnesium. You need certain minerals and vitamins to stay healthy, and this includes mental and physical health. Magnesium deficiency can cause a number of unpleasant side effects and impact your feelings of overall well-being as it is an imperative mineral that affects your nervous system. Many of these effects can be corrected by magnesium supplements.

Magnesium is a crucial dietary element that helps maintain the health of your nervous system. It has an inhibitory effect on the brain chemicals that are responsible for signaling transmission between nerve cells, also known as neurotransmitters.

Magnesium especially helps with the manufacturing of dopamine, which has a primary function of providing a calming effect on your brain. Foods that can increase production of dopamine include nuts, tofu, green, and leafy veggies and beans.

Nervous System Hyperexcitability

Nervous system hyperexcitability also known as Neuromyotonia causes spontaneous straining of your muscles. This hyperexcitability is due to magnesium deficiency and can develop differently depending on age, wear, and gender. An increase in sodium conductance is also caused by magnesium deficiency, which concerns the nervous system because increased sodium conductance results in over-activity that affects both the central as well as the peripheral nervous systems.

With a lack of magnesium, muscles become hyperexcitable (they tend to work more and aggressively), which can make them more responsive to noxious stimuli. This means that you will spend more energy and muscle power on a particular task than needed.

If you have hyperexcitability then you also will have an increased activity of dopamine, aspartate, acetylcholine, glutamate, and norepinephrine. There is a simultaneous decrease in the activity of inhibitory neuromodulators that shape daily life functions responsible for passing information from one neuron to another.

People respond slowly and are lazy if there is a decrease in neuromodulators. These modulators include GABA, melatonin, serotonin, and taurine. Melatonin requires adequate magnesium for proper regulation. Irregularity equates to sleep complications arising and overflowing into daytime fatigue.

Your body has numerous compensatory mechanisms that allow magnesium deficiency to go undetected. This makes you unaware and leads to the development of 'latent nervous system hyperexcitability.' When a patient has low magnesium levels prior to the development of symptoms, he will already be magnesium deficient (even before the symptoms show up). How this nervous system hyperexcitability develops in a person is unknown, although hyperexcitable muscles and frequenting chiropractors will result.

So you should not be surprised that magnesium deficiency is a cause of heterogeneous disease in humans. What to do? - Of course, same as before, increase your intake of magnesium. This can include any sources from the lists mentioned already.

The Health of Nerves

Even a child knows that he needs vitamin C for healthy gums, plenty of protein for muscles, and calcium for strong bones. On the other hand ask the same child or even an adult what foods are good for his nerves, and chances are that he will not know. Fortunately, the proteins, fats, and vitamins are plenty in the average diet. However one nutrient, whose lack may be the cause, and one has been found to be lacking in the diets of most people, and the ultimate cause of nervous illness, is magnesium.

Research shows that electronic measuring techniques have been used to study the electrical conduction of current by the nerves. The findings indicated that magnesium maintains the normal levels of calcium in the nervous system, though it is calcium that acts as the prime conduction of these minute electrical currents.

How Does Magnesium Regulate Calcium Levels?

Inside the body, calcium and magnesium are positively charged. An electric current is formed when these two minerals come into contact with negatively charged particles. Fatty acids that comprise the larger portion of nerve tissue are negatively charged. It is for this reason that magnesium and calcium supplies must be constantly renewed by eating magnesium-rich foods or else the flow of current by the nerve tissues cannot be maintained.

For example, positive and negative electrodes are present to maintain electrical current in a storage battery. The battery is no longer useful if the positive plates become exhausted. Using this same mechanism, you should understand that, a small amount of electrical current flows from calcium ions to the negatively charged nerve lipids. The nerve cells cease to function if there is the absence of adequate calcium. Calcium is not enough because magnesium levels are low, and so the calcium supply becomes exhausted.

Calms the Nerves

Other than proper functioning of the nerve tissues, magnesium also helps to preserve the health of the nervous system. During the early nineteen twenties, doctors were able to learn that magnesium injections act like a depressant effect upon the nerves. In fact, magnesium was used to induce sleep in patients suffering from insomnia (lack of sleep). In fact, high magnesium levels are significant in hibernating animals.

Magnesium has also been shown to be effective in controlling ‘the shakes’ in alcoholics, epileptic seizures and convulsions in pregnant women. The paradoxical effect of this mineral is that if a person with low magnesium levels takes magnesium then he/she feels more energetic than before, even though it is not a stimulant, but a depressant. Magnesium relieves the excessive energy and nervous irritability which can give rise to fatigue in the first place.

When a person’s magnesium levels are subnormal, then you should not be surprised that the nerves are unable to control functions such as mental processes, muscle movement, and respiration. Some symptoms that are due to magnesium-nerve relation and magnesium depletion are twitching, irritability, nervous fatigue, and irregular heartbeat. Coexisting illnesses, such as intestinal infection can cause impairment of absorption of minerals. In such a case, the absorbed magnesium may get lost from the body.

A Host of Disorders

In a recent study, it was shown how an inadequate amount of magnesium coupled with gastrointestinal loss causes a host of nerve disorders. For a better understanding, consider an example that took place in New York in June 1965:

A 28-year-old man was having severe intestinal trouble for the past six years and finally had significant portions of his small and large colon removed. After a period of seven months, he was again admitted to the hospital for a broken vertebra which resulted from a generalized convulsion that shook his body during sleep. On extensive questioning from the family, it was noted that he used to be mildly confused at times and was increasingly irritable. He also used to have twitching of the face, hands, muscles, and feet.

Later on, he suffered from a second convulsion that left him 'agitated', 'anxious', and 'shattered.' His pulse was double the average (70) beats per minute. A dose of magnesium sulfate was injected into his body. His neuromuscular and restlessness problems ceased and overall disappeared! Over time, his need for magnesium gradually diminished as his bowel functions improved. [13]

Another example is how magnesium deficient animals develop neurological damage. When cattle cannot obtain enough magnesium in large amounts from chlorophyll (the green color matter in grass), grass tetany (a metabolic disease involving magnesium deficiency) results. Frothing at the mouth, increased pulse rate, muscle spasms, and fatal convulsions occur due to prolonged magnesium depletion. Sometimes magnesium levels drop to the point that continuous massive doses of magnesium are required.

Due to the severity of the condition, magnesium should not always be taken because overdoses of magnesium can cause profound depression to the entire nervous system and ultimately paralysis of the respiratory system.

The possibility of this danger may increase when a woman in her pregnancy stage develops preeclampsia (A potentially dangerous complication of pregnancy characterized by high blood pressure).

About one in 500 pregnant women suffer from this condition and usually have symptoms such as dizziness, convulsions, headaches, and nausea.

In such cases, the placenta delivers harmful chemical substances in products or blood to the fetus because the body is unable to properly excrete these toxins due to a lack of magnesium. It has almost become a precautionary measure for hospitals to inject the mother with magnesium to facilitate kidney function and control eclamptic convulsions.

The basis of magnesium for the nervous system still requires further research and evidence. However, from the above results, you can be sure that unless your body is satisfactory with ample magnesium, your nervous system can degenerate severely.

A good diet that contains meat, nuts, vegetables and fruits can help lessen the chances of developing several nervous disorders that can stem from a magnesium imbalance.

What Your Medicine Box Needs

There is a high probability that your doctor does not know every role that magnesium plays, nor its indispensability in your general health and metabolism. The fact is; researchers make new discoveries every day. Moreover, it is becoming more apparent that magnesium is one of the most basic nutrients to your health.

Epilepsy, a disorder in that the nerve cell activity in the brain is disturbed, causes seizures. This disease has remained the great mystery of medicine. While hundreds and thousands of other illnesses are treatable, epilepsy remains one of the incurable disorders.

However, research suggests that lower magnesium levels in the spinal fluid may be a cause of epilepsy. If administered properly magnesium can be expected to bring about quick improvement. Current reports hold that subsequent effects on major and minor nerves of the spine running to and from the brain could be due to a deficiency in magnesium, thus actually causing epilepsy.

Deficiency Caused Convulsions

A recent study showed that, a newborn infant developed convulsions due to a metabolic abnormality that did not allow the child to utilize its magnesium absorption correctly. On three tries, the decrease or withdrawal of magnesium supplements led to a fall in both plasma-calcium and plasma-magnesium levels. This caused a reestablishment of the convulsions. If the nervous system is deprived of adequate magnesium, then your entire body will be affected. [14]

Motor nerves (the ones used to carry messages from the brain to the muscles by the effect of stimuli) are likewise dependent on magnesium for proper conduction of these minute electrical messages.

Add to this the essentiality of the same mineral for hard healthy teeth and bones, "and for the functioning of many of our enzyme systems, and we believe it becomes evident that a person would have to be a fool to take any chance on not getting enough magnesium for even a single day." [15]

Chapter 8: Magnesium and Bones

You know that potassium is necessary for bones and helps inhibits osteoporosis, but did you know that magnesium also plays an indispensable role for healthy bones? People with higher magnesium levels have stronger bones and higher bone density than compared to people with low magnesium levels.

Numerous arthritis patients have demineralized bone, so it would benefit them to include a lot of magnesium in their diet, as magnesium is critical for bone mineralization. Magnesium assures the firmness and strength of the bones, while at the same time makes teeth strong and hard. Magnesium plays an important role together with the parathyroid and thyroid glands in supporting bone health. It does so by regulating the parathyroid hormone (whose function is to govern bone breakdown in a myriad of ways) and stimulating the thyroid production of calcitonin, which acts as a bone-preserving hormone.

"Most people are aware that we need to get enough calcium to protect and strengthen our bones and teeth, but fewer people know that magnesium is also vital. About half the magnesium in our body is stored in the bones – it is a constituent of the bone crystals. Therefore, if you are taking a calcium supplement, it may well be worth adding a magnesium supplement as well, to achieve a better balance."[3] For creating an abundance of calcium in the body, there should be abundant magnesium.

Essentials of Magnesium

A vital factor in 80 percent of all cellular enzymes, magnesium is necessary for the conversion of vitamin D into its active form. A syndrome known as vitamin D resistance is seen due to deficiency of magnesium. Alkaline Phosphatase is an enzyme that is required for forming new calcium crystals. It also requires magnesium for triggering and activating it, and if your magnesium levels are low then abnormal bone crystal formation may occur.

As with calcium, 60 percent of the body's reserve of magnesium is held in the bones. Bones act as a storage tank, where transferring of magnesium into the blood stream is needed from time to time. Adequate levels of magnesium are critical throughout life to keep the magnesium that is stored in your body from depleting.

Chapter 9: List of Disorders

The following is a list of common disorders associated with magnesium and how to prevent them:

1. **Insomnia**: Insomnia, also known as lack of sleep is often caused by magnesium deficiency. Magnesium calms your nerves. If you are deficient, then your sympathetic nervous system and heart rate is sent into overdrive. Additionally, it has been shown to alter electrical activity in the brain that causes frequent awakening and agitated sleep. People with poor sleep quality, when given magnesium supplements, have shown improved sleep quality. *Tip: Take magnesium before sleeping, maybe 1/2 a cup of spinach juice to de-stress.*

2. **Dysfunctions of the Brain**: Magnesium regulates a key receptor that supports learning and memory. Decreased brain electrical activity has been seen in people with low magnesium levels. For maintaining the plasticity of synapses, adequate magnesium content in the cerebrospinal fluid is essential. Magnesium is used for the proper activity of many enzymes within brain cells that control memory and cellular functions. *Tip: Magnesium improves your memory and makes your brain work better. For exceptional memory, magnesium is essential.*

3. **Depression**: Magnesium affects the particular neurotransmitters responsible for the discharge of serotonin (a brain chemical that can make an individual feel good). It helps in preventing a chronic low mood and depression.

4. **Low Muscle and Testosterone Levels**: Magnesium is necessary for physical performance and energy metabolism. New research shows that deficiency in magnesium can cause a decline in athletic health and testosterone levels. When combined with exercise, magnesium supplementation raises testosterone levels; which in turn enhances physical performance. *Tip: You are missing out on muscle gain and peak performance if you are not optimizing your magnesium storages.*

5. **Minimum and Weak Protein Synthesis**: Magnesium supports synthesis of proteins in the body as it enables enzyme function in the body. When paired with resistance exercise, magnesium supplementation can make you stronger. *Tip: For muscle development, optimize magnesium levels.*

6. **A Decrease in Heart Health/ Increase in Inflammation**: Inflammation is not only an obstacle that you face after hard workouts, but it is also responsible for heart diseases, diabetes, arthritis, and Alzheimer's. Magnesium deficiency leads to increase in inflammation in the body which affects, cardiovascular tissues, blood vessels, and the intestinal tissues. A deficiency in magnesium also increases blood pressure and decreases lipid metabolism, which acts as a negative impact on the health of your arteries, causing atherosclerosis. *Tip: In order to reduce inflammation, take magnesium. It is critical for cardiovascular health.*

7. **Weak Bones**:

Osteoporosis: Vitamin D and calcium are necessary for stronger bones, but it is to no avail if you do not have adequate levels of magnesium. Bone building and calcium absorption can be done by converting vitamin D to its active form, which can be done only by magnesium. Magnesium releases the hormone calcitonin, which helps to draw calcium out of the blood and soft tissue, and also preserves the bone structure. *Tip: Without adequate magnesium, a calcium supplement is useless. Combine magnesium and calcium in equal doses, and don't forget to add vitamin D.*

8. **Diabetes**: Low magnesium levels decrease your insulin sensitivity, which in turn makes it harder for you to get lean and lose fat. A longer recovery from workouts will result as the body's storage of glycogen is disturbed. Poorly controlled diabetes and increased insulin resistance result in more magnesium loss. *Tip: Including magnesium in your diet can prevent diabetes and supports a lean body composition.*

9. **Metabolic Syndrome/Magnesium and Pregnancy**: Low magnesium levels are common in pregnancy and are a risk to the further development of diabetes and may cause Metabolic Syndrome in the child after birth. Metabolic syndrome is an inflammatory condition, and lack of magnesium can cause oxidative stress and inflammation to the sympathetic nervous system. *Tip: Eat magnesium-rich foods.*

10. **Stress**: Low magnesium levels can affect norepinephrine release and the nervous system, which causes stress and worry. In order to return to a relaxed state faster, magnesium is essential for the metabolism of cortisol. *Tip: Cortisol is lowered by healthy magnesium levels.*

11. **Digestive-Related Diseases and Constipation**: There are many symptoms of magnesium deficiency concerning digestion. They include: Fatigue, muscle tremors and twitching, irritability, reduced mental function, and insomnia. Magnesium affects the gastrointestinal tract, allowing proper functioning while improving digestion. *Tip: High levels of magnesium eliminate constipation and improve digestion. This lowers colon cancer risk and diabetes.*

Magnesium and Your Diet

Six Ways You Can Increase Your Magnesium Levels:

[The methods listed below will help you alleviate hormonal symptoms]

1. Eat dark chocolate that consists of 80% of cocoa in moderation. The less sugar it contains, the more magnesium you get. *Dark chocolate contains more magnesium than any other food source*. Eighty percent or more cocoa are present in dark chocolate.

2. Eat magnesium-rich food: nuts, seeds, burdock root, leafy greens, nettles and whole grains. Other sources- by milligrams per 3-1/2 ounces- include: Wheat germ (336); Kelp (760); Buckwheat (229); wheat bran (490); cashews (267) and dulse (220)

3. **Reduce "magnesium suckers"**: Processed foods, exposure to environmental toxins, high alcohol consumption, smoking, and stress.

4. **Snack** on sunflower seeds and pumpkin seeds (or their butters).

5. **Take supplemental magnesium**, such as magnesium citrate powder. In 16 ounces of water mix two rounded teaspoons of magnesium citrate, and keep sipping slowly throughout the day. Again in the evening, you should drink the same drink in the same proportions.

6. **Epsom salt soaks**: In two quarts of warm water, dissolve 1 cup of Epsom salts for a foot soak. For a bath mix 2 cups of Epsom salts. Soak for 25 to 30 minutes

Ways to Boost Your Energy

What foods do you eat to keep your daily dose of magnesium derived energy consistent?

Magnesium Intake: For ensuring that your mineral and vitamin needs are met you should eat a balanced diet. For making sure that you get enough magnesium acquired energy, include into your diet: hazelnuts, cashews or almonds, bran cereal, and whole grains. Eating more fish also helps, especially halibut.

Additional foods that can increase your magnesium levels are: wheat germ, kelp, collard greens, filberts, tofu, soy beans, dandelion greens, shrimp, parsley, garlic, pecans, buckwheat, millet, Brazil nuts, avocados, and peas.

Throughout the day, consuming any five of these magnesium-rich foods can help you maintain your energy levels. They include:

1 cup of brown rice
1/2 cup of boiled spinach
1 cup of raisin bran
1/2 cup of quinoa
1 cup of oatmeal
1 cup of kidney beans
1 cup of lentils
2 bananas
1 cup of shredded wheat
2 slices of whole wheat bread

How Much Magnesium Does Your Body Require?

You should ask your doctor for a magnesium red blood test which is used to measure magnesium levels. It usually ranges from 4.3 to 6.7—the optimal level is 6.5. So, if you are below 6.0, you are magnesium deficient.

Magnesium Supplements: The minimum amount of magnesium needed for a healthy adult is about 300 mg, but most of us consume less than 200 mg! Depending on the individual's condition, others may require more (some more than 1000 mg per day).

NEW BONUS CHAPTER:

The Best Forms of Magnesium!

As is known, there are MANY forms of magnesium. Purchasing the 'right one' becomes that much more difficult of a decision to make when there are so many to choose from. There is not necessarily a form that is 'best' per se, but there are forms that are more readily absorbed and offer different benefits due to the molecule it is bonded to.

For example, magnesium malate is bonded with malic acid which promotes ATP synthesis resulting in more energy, less fatigue, and helps with fibromyalgia. It is important to consult your doctor to help you decide which type might be best suitable for your body specifically.

In general the best oral form is chelated because it is more readily absorbed into the system. The common form that tends to be non-chelated is oxide. Oxide usually contains elemental magnesium that, rather than being absorbed, gets stuck in the gut until it is flushed out.

The Best Bioavailable Forms are:

Magnesium Threonate- *NEW* may be the best currently on the market

Magnesium Oratate- great for more serious deficiency (high absorption)

Magnesium Taurate- great for heart health

Magnesium Glycinate- great for individuals prone to loose stools

Magnesium Malate or dimalate – great for energy

Magnesium Citrate- great for individuals prone to constipation

Magnesium Chloride- great for metabolism and detoxing cells

Can I Take Multiple Forms?

Yes, in fact, many doctors will recommend taking magnesium in a variety of its forms.
Glycinate, orotate, citrate, and taurinate are four that have been recommended to take in combination by Dr Sinatra.

Most Popular:

Magnesium citrate, known to be on the lesser expensive end, is popular and a good choice for absorption. Powder form is preferred for this type.

Worst Forms:

Magnesium oxide- contains high amounts of elemental magnesium and is poorly absorbed

Magnesium sulfate- easily overdosed

Magnesium glutamate- a neurotoxin if not bound to amino acids

Magnesium aspartate- a neurotoxin if not bound to amino acids

Common Forms That Cause Diarrhea:

Magnesium carbonate, Magnesium chloride, magnesium gluconate, and magnesium oxide

Heart Health:

Magnesium taurate is recommended for people who have cardiovascular problems. Magnesium taurate is the magnesium combined with taurine. Taurine is an amino acid (one of the 9 essential amino acids) that stabilizes the membranes of cells, making magnesium able to be absorbed.

Taurine is crucial for heart health and can be used as a preventative measure against heart damage associated with heart attacks as well as arrhythmia.

When to Supplement it:

Take magnesium once in the morning and once before bed. The water solubility of magnesium (every form) will require this morning and night routine. However, over-supplementation is possible. Follow dietary daily allowance guidelines and consult your primary doctor should you have any questions.

Magnesium and Antibiotics

Magnesium does have reactions with some antibiotics. If you are newly considering taking magnesium, but are already on antibiotics it is important to check with your doctor. The timeframes between supplementing magnesium and taking your regular antibiotic may need a 2-4 hour window in between. Information regarding supplementation should not take the place of medical advice.

Quick Favor Please…

If you liked this book, please take a moment to leave a review on Amazon letting me know if you have learned from this book.

I always want to hear from my readers and know how your healthy life style is going.
Thank You and Good Luck

Bibliography

Azoulay A, Garzon P, Eisenberg MJ. Comparison of the mineral content of tap water and bottled waters. J Gen Intern Med 2001;16:168-75. [PubMed abstract]

Calcium vs. magnesium: The key is balance | PCC Natural Markets. (n.d.). Retrieved from http://www.pccnaturalmarkets.com/sc/0403/sc0403-expertadv.html [1]

Did You Know Magnesium contributes to the health of bones and ... (n.d.). Retrieved from http://www.nutricentre.com/healthsupplementsblog/2013/07/did-you-know-magnesium/ [3]

Elin RJ. Assessment of magnesium status for diagnosis and therapy.Magnes Res 2010;23:1-5. [PubMed abstract]

Fisherman, Dr Robert. Archives of Neurology (June, 1965). New York[13]

Fine KD, Santa Ana CA, Porter JL, Fordtran JS. Intestinal absorption of magnesium from food and supplements. J Clin Invest 1991;88:396-402. [PubMed abstract]

Gibson, RS. Principles of Nutritional Assessment, 2nd ed. New York, NY: Oxford University Press, 2005.

http://www.wellnessresources.com/health/articles/the_five_key_things_you_can_do_to_lower_ldl_cholesterol_healthfully/

Institute of Medicine (IOM).Food and Nutrition Board. Dietary Reference Intakes: Calcium, Phosphorus, Magnesium, Vitamin D and Fluorideexternal link icon. Washington, DC: National Academy Press, 1997.

Insulin Sensitivity – Diabetes.(n.d.). Retrieved from http://www.diabetes.co.uk/insulin/insulin-sensitivity.html[6]

Magnesium and Heart Health - Heart Health Center - Everyday ...(n.d.). Retrieved from http://www.everydayhealth.com/heart-health-specialist/magnesium.aspx [2]

Magnesium and muscle performance in older persons: the ... (n.d.). Retrieved from http://ajcn.nutrition.org/content/84/2/419.full [11]

Magnesium | DrDeborahMD.com.(n.d.). Retrieved from http://www.drdeborahmd.com/magnesium [8]

Magnesium requirements: new estimations for men and women by ... (n.d.). Retrieved from http://ajcn.nutrition.org/content/84/4/843.abstract[7]

Magnesium, The Nutrient That Could Change Your Life: Chapter ... (n.d.). Retrieved from http://www.mgwater.com/rod06.shtml [12, 14, 15]

Magnesium: This Invisible Deficiency Can Harm Your Health. (n.d.). Retrieved from http://articles.mercola.com/sites/articles/archive/2015/01/19/magnesium-deficiency.aspx

McDonald R1, Keen CL (1988). Iron, zinc and magnesium nutrition and athletic performance, Sports Med.; 5(3): 171-84.[10]

Nadler JL, Buchanan T, Natarajan R, Antonipillai I, Bergman R, Rude R: Magnesium deficiency produces insulin resistance and increased thromboxane synthesis. Hypertension 21:1024–1029, 1993 [4]

Natural Strategies For Lowering Cholesterol | Dr Briffa's ... (n.d.). Retrieved from http://www.drbriffa.com/2001/09/11/natural-strategies-for-lowering-cholesterol/[5]

Number of Children with Vitamin D Deficiency Soars. (n.d.). Retrieved from http://articles.mercola.com/sites/articles/archive/2014/11/10/vitamin-d-deficien [9]

Rude RK.Magnesium. In: Coates PM, Betz JM, Blackman MR, Cragg GM, Levine M, Moss J, White JD, eds. Encyclopedia of Dietary Supplements. 2nd ed. New York, NY: Informa Healthcare; 2010:527-37.

Rude RK.Magnesium. In: Ross AC, Caballero B, Cousins RJ, Tucker KL, Ziegler TR, eds. Modern Nutrition in Health and Disease. 11th ed. Baltimore, Mass: Lippincott Williams & Wilkins; 2012:159-75.

Volpe SL. Magnesium. In: Erdman JW, Macdonald IA, Zeisel SH, eds. Present Knowledge in Nutrition. 10th ed. Ames, Iowa; John Wiley & Sons, 2012:459-74.

Witkowski M, Hubert J, Mazur A. Methods of assessment of magnesium status in humans: a systematic review. Magnesium Res 2011;24:163-80. [PubMed abstract]

U.S. Department of Agriculture, Agricultural Research Service. USDA National Nutrient Database for Standard Reference, Release 25. Nutrient Data Laboratory Home Pageexternal link icon, 2012

Printed in Great Britain
by Amazon

65246180R00047

SPLINTERING THE DARK

Also by Wendy French

Sky Over Bedlam
(tall lighthouse press)

We Have A Little Sister And She Hath No Breasts
(tall lighthouse press)

Wendy French

Wendy

Splintering the Dark

Elizabeth –
good to meet
you at poetry!
August 2012

Rockingham Press

Published in 2005 by
The Rockingham Press
11 Musley Lane,
Ware, Herts SG12 7EN
www.rockinghampress.com

British Library Cataloguing-in-Publication Data

A catalogue record for this book
is available from the British Library

ISBN 1 904851 03 7

Printed in Great Britain
by Biddles Limited
King's Lynn

ARTS COUNCIL ENGLAND

for my sister Diane
and
in memory of my niece Rachael (1977-2003)

With special thanks to William who is my rock;
my sons Ben and Tom, who with Nikki and Rebecca
have brought me laughter and tears
and to my parents who continue to show courage.
Thanks also to Anne-Marie Fyfe for friendship and
inspiration, Dilys Wood for selfless encouragement and
David Perman for his help in publishing two anthologies
of poetry for hospital schools and for this book.

CONTENTS

Acknowledgements

Acknowledgments are due to the editors of the following publications in which some of these poems first appeared: *Magma, Spokes, Tears in the Fence, The Interpreter's House, Acumen, Smiths Knoll, Foolscap, Ivor Gurney Society Journal, The Wolf* and *Poetry Nottingham.*

"Sea" appeared in *Oxfam Competition Anthology*, "The Therapist Talks Back" appeared in the *Berkshire Competition Anthology*. "Lunch-Time" appeared in *Ware Competition Anthology.*

Anthologies: "Voyez-vous cet Oeuf", "CT Scan", "African Horizons"and "Graffiti" appeared in *Four Caves of The Heart.* "Swimming towards the Flow", "Olga" and "Mauritshuis" appeared in *Entering the Tapestry.*

The roses tremble; oh, the sunflower's eye
Is opened wide in sad expectancy.

Denise Levertov

SKY OVER BEDLAM

It dawned on me as we stared
up past roofs into walls climbing the sky
overlooking the significance of motorways
that we might all be drowning in the morning.

LUNCH-TIME

With forty-five minutes to spare
I step out of the asylum
pass redbrick pillars
shielding silence.

Not hungry I stop
to explore shelves
of books to be borrowed or thumbed.
The librarian checks me up and down as I open
a selected copy on psychosis, its musty theories divorced
from the world
                                        of Sam
who, dehydrated, sits with his feet in a bowl of water.

Concentration is needed to coil a pot
                                        the kiln fires as he sits
with a basin containing two size tens.

I close the book, place it in its rightful slot
amble through the electronic gate, swing through doors
to rain-drenched branches of trees in spring blossom.
Men are drilling pavements, laying cables
to connect one person to another.

There's no alternative but to turn
                                    back under colluding skies
to a staff-room
                    where coffee percolates.

CT SCAN

We sit on the mini bus and tell stories
to pass the time
but you can't move on – your thoughts
are stuck, thinking about the slipper
that fitted Cinderella. You want
to go back to the ward; you're nervous
and that makes me edgy.

I try to start a new story, one to enjoy
but you make me repeat Cinderella
word for word, starting with the death
of a mother; this time, the fairy godmother's
the health visitor, anorexic Cinderella
wants to live in the cellar refusing bread,
working the pounds off, up and down stairs.
Some prince will rescue you
from this death you are leading us to.

You take off your trainers, examine your size 6
and in a second the shoe's
through the window. You watch
to see who'll retrieve it
as the driver negotiates London traffic
to reach your appointment on time.

ROOF GARDEN

You step onto the roof
the out-of-bounds, gasp

as the garden is revealed, you dig
a hole wide enough to take a hawthorn tree.

Dust to dust, you say
and ask me to remove my top.

We need to show we're sane.
You admire the headless stork

overlooking a parched pond
where lilies opened once.

There is an underworld
of moistures deep in a roof garden.

WHEN THE WATERS BREAK

On your sixtieth
a daughter sings happy birthday
down the phone.

Looking at the 5 a.m. digital
you aren't surprised
when the call ends abruptly

and she screams *Not many more now.*
When her acute phase
has passed, you accept the diagnosis

of schizophrenia, and drink
bottle after bottle of cheap
red wine, but in the dawn

when once your waters broke
words hand you back an emptiness
it's difficult to grieve for.

BIRD SONG

I sleep in the corner of morning.
Fly without wings through the ward.
Beyond the window the sun breaks
over rhododendrons. A man
with a fish stands alone looking
for a God seen running with the bread
embroidered on tapestry woven in therapy.

White roses and fern stem from the carpet.
The psychiatrist's dream is his vocation.
He weeds thoughts, plucks dandelions
bends double to digest words
that escape from my mouth.
In the past red wine loosened my tongue
lithium now leaves it dry.

His trousers match my skirt. Charity-shop shoes
give freedom to dance. The always-other world
excitedly here. Every morning I tell them my stories
they increase medication. Steal
my dreams. Write them up in their notes.
Lock another door.
Throw cake to the parakeets.

WHITE IS NOT AN ABSENCE

William Blake

And in she comes with her multi-coloured strands
twirling a Japanese umbrella high above her head
as she waltzes, one-two-three, one-two-three
weaving in and out of dilapidated library desks
where distracted minds try hard to scan patterns in Blake.
Her animated bodies smile, kick back their chairs and join
in earth's dance. One sings *I'm a fruit and nut case*

and everyone forgets the poet to pick up the beat
of the blues. She wears the mask of the god
that she wants us to believe in. And the words
leap off the page as white becomes anything
but an absence in her presence, as her mind
one step ahead, persuades her to call the tune
in the absence, not of white, but of yesterday's medication.

SWIMMING TOWARDS THE FLOW

He didn't know your history;
hadn't skimmed your notes.
Said he preferred to imagine you a fresh
young eel swimming against the tide.
He handed you a pair of ill-fitting trunks
and you proclaimed, *Like swim, like swim*
and stepping in confidently
disappeared to the bottom.

A sleepy afternoon, the alert lifeguard
was with you in seconds and you rolled
and coughed on the slippery side
as youngsters sniggered. In Somalia
there are no signs warning of danger.
Written up clinically, a vivid description
of the night the police pulled you in
cold against the pull of the Thames

struggling against water and uniforms.
Weeping, your father later translated
that the white angels of heaven floated upstream
and enticed you to join them, flaunting
a message that was held tantalisingly
just to the right of your life.

THE CONCERT PIANIST

for years
he played faithfully this b minor
                he now taps on the windowsill
memories that grew with him

ebony-finished steinways
iron wrought balconies champagne in intervals

bow-ties
his mother's smile
           looking up from her piano
and her photograph
always and still
         next to his bed

too young to understand
when she'd left he'd been content
with letters
              envelopes

coloured stamps koala bears

but now this chord
always this chord (she'd played over and over again)
haunts his waking dreams
his sleeping hours

and tomorrow
two male nurses
                 will accompany him
as the minister takes him to the chapel and as it is easter

he will be
  triumphant allowed to play

passing through a mist of empty flower beds
this open walk will lead him

                                        to a god who listens to voices imitate
the sane and he will deliver a chopin prelude to a captive congre-
gation

who choose shuffling from locked wards to this resurrection
and days echoing that first cold morning

THE THERAPIST TALKS BACK

Talking to you is like screwing down a coffin lid
or carrying water in cupped hands
across the desert. I've never known you not to cheat
but face to face you never tell a lie, and this

is like carrying water in cupped hands.
That's how hard it was to try and reach you
but face to face you never tell a lie.
You just hid the tablets till we were out of sight.

That's how hard it was to try and reach you.
If you'd survived the weekend it would have been all right.
You just hid the tablets till we were out of sight.
In the ambulance you'd asked if you were going to die.

If you'd survived the weekend it would have been all right.
A nurse telephoned to say that she'd been with you when you died.
In the ambulance you'd asked if you were going to die.
In our last session you'd seemed to want to live.

A nurse telephoned to say that she'd been with you when you died.
Across the desert I've never known you not to cheat.
In our last session you'd seemed to want to live.
Talking to you is like screwing down a coffin lid.

MESSAGE

The night you killed yourself the duty nurse phoned.
She swore she'd left a message on my machine.

So after I'd heard officially, replaying my messages –
your voice – *You say the day. I'll be there.*

The summer exhibition or Brighton Rock at the ICA.
I can't decide; I'm taken with smoke filled clouds

travelling aimlessly across pure cold and pale skies.

NEW EVERY MORNING

I go down to the music cells
watch your hands slide
over music that was speaking to you
even before hands touched the notes
every day the piece sounded
triumphant or down-beat
Greensleeves Fantasia you always started with
and thirty five years later I still hear you
see you in that unbecoming uniform clinging
to your breasts your national health glasses
that needed cleaning every day after I'd left your bed
before prefects did room-check so we wouldn't
be punished for being young away from home
but I can't say homesick because you gave me
a friendship that I hadn't known existed
you helped me touch the keys
and you persevered because you believed
I could do it so you tried to teach me
but in the end there wasn't time so I only learnt
some tune to do with the sea
and every time I stand on the cliffs at Pendine
whether it's summer or nearly summer
and the children are laughing or nearly laughing
I can't believe that I was ever as young as that
because too quickly one morning we weren't
fast enough and were discovered and the word pervert
still smarts as your specs blurred with tears
and my paralysed stammer fixed on the frothing foam
resting on the prefect's words

we lost touch and now I've read in the newsletter you're not there
anymore so I traced your parents you'd stopped eating
and slit your wrists and then you overdosed
and I couldn't ask too many questions
but I'm still desperate to know how did they find you
and did they leave your glasses on as you were lowered
down

OBSESSION

for Ivor Gurney

I wake in the early hours
flounder for sense
but it's you again –

looking back
at the camera. Eyes pierce me.
Suit falls off a skeleton frame.

The photographic image
imprinted on my brain
archives 49 – archives 49.

Day out with Marion.
You're still in the asylum
but with me each day.

Your limbs shake with fear
threatened by electricity.
I'm trying to talk to you

to hand you agapanthus,
to ask about line-ends
to hear about Scott

discuss Edward Thomas
to touch you before you escape.
Hurl yourself again into my madness.

When the journey's over
There'll be time enough to sleep.

A.E. Housman

DUNGENESS

Hesitations of a summer ending.
Smoke from wood-burning stoves
and a feeling this is the end of the world
where nets are mended, small boats turn out to sea.

AFRICAN HORIZONS

In a school in Dekeza, we leave books, pens.
Elizabeth Bishop sits on a library shelf –

the edition with a cover of blue skies
darker seas, white boat, red maple leaves.

Without need for language
a hungry boy cries for a bowl of sadza.

Ghosts of starvation holler through trees.
Listen to the sound that comes from sorrow –

sorrow lights up under a full moon
it floods the fields, dying crops.

Children play on the edge
where leopards come.

A red country green in its unrest.
Tensions burn underground.

But the president wears a coat of one colour.
His country is his coat; we allow him to wear it.

I am a woman whose muted protest knits Mugabe
into the sleeve of a cashmere coat.

THE GARDEN

You touch the baby's cheek
and make her cry.
She's used to women bending
watering the green in a dried earth
where cattle graze thinly.

All day women wait.
Wait for a turn at the water pump.
Wait on a red land to fill carriers
while children play and men hang
round the bottle store, sing
sacred songs for scud.

All night women lie down.
Lie down for men who have been singing
while they've been tending the garden.

SEE YOU

Along a brown-red earth a boy walks.
He seems to have come from nowhere
but knows how far he has to go.

He swings a bag, hoping for a lift
but not expecting one.
Sundown is hours away.

There's life in his shoes.
His belly is empty but with luck
there will be sadza enough for evening.

More water makes it go further.
He thinks of his mother bending over a fire
stirring her hips in rhythm with the spoon.

It's Friday and school's out.
A car stops and takes him forty kilometres.
See you he says as he runs for the fields.

MAURITSHUIS

for William: February 1996

Snow melting our faces
we left all those Vermeers
behind locked doors – this time

we were too early. Hands frozen
together we hid disappointments
in woolly gloves.

You rationalised feelings
and said anyway we'd seen
most of them before

and then you danced along cobbles
to make me laugh
pretending you were drunk

riding a bicycle into the Hofvijver.
And all I wanted was The View of the Delft;
the lady reading the letter.

SWEET CHESTNUTS

We have come here before
feel safe in humidity of palms
climb spiral steps, from balconies
we gaze at the huge ambivalence
of tropical plants – butterflies
balanced on the edge and we talk
about the delicacy of daily lives.
When we're home we'll savour
the brightness of that summer day
the display of medicinal herbs.
How time is not a healer.

I'll memorise the words –
catch-phrases fall like beads of sweat
slates of the Fern House floor reflect
a cool drizzle from the past. Convince me
that by tomorrow's shade we'll think
of remedies we've nurtured
the passion flower that flourishes
in cherished climates but most of all
how sweet chestnuts are pulped
into a juice to be swallowed down
when it seems no light is left.

WAITING IN AMSTERDAM

He wandered through the house, looking.
Studying in depth etching after etching
gazing past Rembrandt into a street
he imagines he hears his daughter enter.

Thoughts for long-gone days haunted
his search in vain through dead canals
and lists of other people's making.
Vermeer's interiors shook visions
as children dance on eggs around a table.

WALLFLOWER

for Rebecca

The woman I once was
wears the wealth on the sleeve
of her gypsy past. I feed her stories
swivel her to face the light.
I planted her in a climate from
Southern Europe so she grew
upright and bloomed early.
Next spring will be hers to flaunt.

In autumn, wallflowers need
little attention. I'll dig my dreams
round her roots. They'll thrive in the wild.

VOYEZ-VOUS CET OEUF

Voyez-vous cet oeuf. C'est avec qu'on renverse toutes
*les écoles du théologie et tous les temples de la terre**
Diderot

The night before he left for Japan
they adapted both their recipes
to spice the henshit-and landmuck-eggs
newly laid that morning.
He washed brown shells with tissue.
She thought she knew his silences.
For the mayonnaise he added one tablespoon
of Dijon mustard. She, the special wine vinegar

to create that tart taste of summer madness.
He cracked the fragile shell
separated white from yolk to whisk
until the salt dissolved. Later, before
leaving, they walked in West Norwood cemetery
searching for Mrs Beeton's grave. She saw
in his eyes a spring of knowledge, something
from his father she'd never seen before.

What guesses did he make about himself?
What about the rejection of every yesterday
that he must feel? She held her breath
for that half-heard affirmative. Dusk comes
creeps into night; hungry by candlelight she searches
the fridge for something cool. Not wanting the tang
of mayonnaise she settles for *oeufs mollets*
whole-meal bread.

**See this egg. It is with this that all the schools of theology and all the temples of the earth are to be overturned.*

CALLING

It's too early to phone
the distance keeps you sleeping
but I press the receiver to my ear
listen for your voice down the line

as if this miracle plastic case
contains the all of you
will bring you nearer
will help you say

the things I want to hear
as if the pretence
of dialling your number
will ignite your dreams

keep them burning 'til morning.
Your night has yet the hope of dawn
and I the insatiable desire to reverse
the universe and speak to you.

OLGA

There were experiences between us
neither could imagine. It was when you said

you couldn't face potato skins because
of the memory of Mama

last seen huddled in a lorry
that it all spilt out. Camps

living in fear, thankful for a skin
clinging to a skirt, thankless for a life.

You looked worn-out
I offered to bake potatoes.

The shudder made me hesitate
I touched your arm.

Opening a bottle of Jack Daniels
it didn't matter that I was young, employed.

You paid three pounds an hour
though half your whiskey was drunk.

We sat telling of lives
lives lit with candles

listening to Wild Man Blues
pasta wound round forks.

Tomorrow you'd go to Chambers
and I'd clean your rooms.

MY ROOM

You may still creep
through my room each morning
to herald thoughts, affect applause.

If, on waking, dreams are realised
then enter my mind
by knocking early at the door.

If I'm not there, step in
quietly not to wake the dead.
I'll be gazing at the misty mirror.

GRAFFITI

Stumbling for a switch, tying a knot
in my Parisian dressing gown, I know
what I'm going to find

three o'clock in the morning. I'm unbolting
the front door with excuses.
They'll be different from yesterday's

and in the porch-light two policemen
are holding you from a night
I don't seem able to.

One is kind, adopts
an absent-father role, pep talks
about the dangers out there.

The other lectures me on child protection
but I'm not listening. I'm travelling
down the Jubilee Line, glueing back

your world, while your window
still hangs open, highlighting your escape
and rain pours in.

SEA

Words in the air, a winter smog
railings worn from rust-eaten years.

We loop the lead of the Labrador through
bent wire. Head for the sands to the sea.

Bach's Prelude plays though the bandstand's
long gone. We sing the tune of the sea as it swims

to shore creating its own sounds
and in the distance behind us

blue has faded down to grey.
What if one day the tide forgets to turn?

WINTER SOLSTICE

She is the furthest from the sun
than she has ever been.
Snow brakes the heavens.
Trees still; skeletons round frozen waters.
In the kitchen she ices cakes. More cakes.

The white runs down the side forming
a lake on the cracked plate
but he will come soon and take her
on the stone floor where the Aga's heat
will warm the curves in her back
and she will sleep till the icing sets.

On top of one cake will be a fir tree.
Green of course.
Different from last year.

PREPARATION

all my skin old age already
(Sappho Fragment 58)

We sat round the wedding guest table
listened to tales of your mother

and how she prepared
her Parma ham. Joints of pig

washed down and salted –
salt rubbed and pulsed

into damp flesh till arms ached
saltpetre preserved cracks of her fingers

and your father carried burdens of meat
high to the Alps, where for a year

they hung under fresh skies, winds and rain sealing
these huge mocking crows that swing the salt.

A present day sacrifice.
Now you lie between white sheets

body transmigrating –
not from cigarettes, you say

but from too much gardening –
you are drawn to the iridescence.

of the night. Look to the stars and see
wild birds soar over mountain edges.

AFTER THE STORM

for Jerry and William

mountain wind falling on oak trees
(Sappho Fragment 95)

How they firm their roots into the ground
grow sideways away from falling rocks

tunnelled soil covers damaged roots
to make a branch whole again. Saplings grow

side by side vying for space to make a height towards the sky.
And now this boy on his bicycle rides

past me in the Elan Valley, observing hills
avoiding roots, this rain-sleeting day

and how he passes sheep sheltering
waves and grins, not knowing who I am

but recognising on this path
a fellow traveller, making me want to weep.

How our perspective changes of a kind or cruel
or impenetrable land.

These oaks, these paths welcome us in to walk
to shelter, observe the contours of a land that tricks us

further in from dark to light and then again to dark.
Sometimes we enter. Follow paths. Search towards the sky.

But a kind of yearning has hold of me.

Sappho Fragment 95

SUNFLOWERS

yes many and beautiful things
(Sappho, Fragment 24)

It is three o'clock on Thursday seventh of August
a sultry heat that dusts the streets with litter –
an unrelenting dryness in the air. I pass a flower-seller
sitting on the step, sunflowers from Israel
fold down into a steel bucket
and then I pause at Van Gogh's sunflowers
newly painted on the outside wall.

Entering the gallery, long corridors protect us
with paintings from unlived centuries
and I find a map to read the way to sunflowers
which dominate and bloom. Outside, I will buy
the sunflowers on offer rather than a postcard
for by morning when they've drooped and died
pollen stains will remain ground into my hearth.

TAKING FLOWERS TO A HOSPITAL BED

I don't know what to do. I'm in two minds
(Sappho Fragment 51)

about whether to buy her daffodils or irises –
the iris does not live for long, but purple petals
fold and match red walls

and though with daffodils in bud
there is the hope of blossoming
bright yellow expectation is too sombre

for her golden hair today.

TO A GOLD EAR-RING

Head of Nefertiti

I conversed with you in a dream
(Sappho Fragment 134)

What I had is lost.
I cannot look at you exactly
but I can talk to you

and I can see and see again
your silted head listening by my ear.
There were two of you – whether in flight

or fall one has disappeared.
I've heard echoes from the past;
how you grew into me, became a part of sleep.

Fourteen years of a straightening
branching out and while the planet
slowly disappears

you will become gold-dust. Ground.
My other ear-ring, carefully removed sits
in a stained glass bowl which reflects my naked face.

WAKING

where are you gone leaving me behind?
(Sappho Fragment 114)

My parents wake the night up.
They hear scratching from the ceiling:
squirrels they say again
turn over, but do not sleep.

No sounds in the morning;
the cat, unperturbed, sleeps on
but on the wall above their heads
a face has loomed.

Paint scraped, two ears
eyes and a mouth that screams
an echo. A Lucien Freud face
exclaims the horrors of collision.

Too thin to survive in daylight
tells news they've heard before.
Dreams trapped in the groove
of an old gramophone record play on.

All day the face stays with them.
In bed they try to pretend they're back
in their first house. The telephone rings
inside their heads, the telephone rings all night.

Gramophone. Telephone – nothing dulls its sound.

LETTER TO DIANE

And her light
Stretches over salt sea
Equally and flowerdeep fields.
(Sappho Fragment 96)

Sometimes before the first star
I lie on my back and wait.
I know she will be sprinting

over hills to catch the dark
to be the first light of night.
I told you it would be this.

Last year's dream and this would come –
the churchyard, Goudhurst – wearing black
and me not able to believe.

The sun shone, I searched the rays
to see the wicker coffin.
In Cranbrook, Chapel of Rest

Rebecca washed Rachael's hair
such long, fair strands glowing
in chilled air. Toes newly

painted, bruised face, gauze neatly
placed over chest drain wounds.
On the pick-your-own sunflower

farm, you, laden with stems, huge
blazing petals for your dead
daughter. Bright pollen falling.

Back in time, children all play.
Rachael rides a hobby horse.
Giddy ups on uneven

ground, stumbles, Rebecca and
her cousins rush forward, soon
Rachael's *hee-hawing*. Tom steals

the toy horse and he gallops
until he falls. Rachael laughs
and so they go on building

a tree-house, swapping conkers.
Plotting. Exploring habitats.
The time we left The Peacock –

she wept said that she loved me
but wouldn't drive back with me.
Over misty New Year fields

she walked home to Flishinghurst.
Your house. A roof you can peer
at the stars through, the children

sit in the fire place, roast nuts.
Warm hands from fishing in the
icy pond. But now she will

not return. The day is fine;
her shadow skips and collects
autumnal leaves, acorns and

pushes into her pocket
tangible objects to covet –
bargain with. Coalitions

are over, this spool gathers some
momentum. Tangles past, present.
For now I sign off Diane.

I will write all our names.

RED SARONG

for Diane

My thinking
not thus
(Sappho Fragment 3)

The delivery man arrives with a bouquet
of well-wishers' thoughts. You kiss him. (What else
on a hot summer day when all is not well?)
You gather loose leaves of Thai silk
into your hands, those flow-freeing folds
red and black and wringing with sweat
from that sultry day as you walk into the house
to replenish the jug with fresh lemon and water.
It's the characteristic hold of your skirt
that confuses for this moment life and death
(who we should kiss)
and just when we are desperately clinging to skirts
someone catches a memory.

MY MOTHER'S COAT

Gather a child to its mother
(Sappho Fragment 104A)

My sister wears my mother's coat
puffed sleeves, A-line *waist drop.*
It suits her well – high collar
with hook and eye and olive green
for autumn days, summer nights.
She wears this coat as she peddles
through lanes shrouded by trees.
She peddles fast, her face clouded
in sunlight. She peddles fast
to convert memories to rhythms
for this day only she wants the past
to dissolve into hedgerows
be picked with blackberries.

WILD DUCKS

Out of the unexpected
(Sappho Fragment 16)

Two wild ducks have settled on the stream
down by the summer house. They flew in one night
and stayed for the storm next day.

What would they say if they could speak?
Not of themselves but where they're from
and how cumbersome the flight.

Would this be comfort? Or is it better not to know
the answers that we seek? How strange
these ducks should settle here when they are needed;

swim round the pond as if familiar with its weeds
its undertones. You feed them not to entice them to danger.
Enough to make them want to stay. They swim as if they know.

They bring some kind of hope, entangled
with an ultimate despair. To dive in unison and then for one
to rise reminds us of the sideways face of death.

THE NEWLY DUG GRAVE

Having been breathed out
(Sappho Fragment 55)

Will we find where –
where petals fold in on flesh
flesh, pink once now white.

The yellow from sunflowers stains
the grass. Colours seep through earth.
A child skips to the edge of the field

to breathe the sky. First breath of the day
for the last breath blew a dandelion to the ground.
At twilight summer will be sung
                                        through trees.

THE YEAR I LEFT SHE DIED

as long as there is in me
(Sappho Fragment 88A)

there's no return

rum thrown over the grave and the impotent calling
sunflowers and a candle from Israel
hills that rise ahead an English Calvary

and the Navy Rum warm in our throats as words blow out –
and the candle incompetent to winter mist and drizzle a hearty
gale preferable to this

we still are buried maybe forever
no longer can guess sweet smells
of dog rose and wonder
if spring will ever come again with daffodils.

The dark an anxious host descends through the churchyard
barren hedges and a distant voice
takes flight retreats

we walk a laborious walk up the steep path

pass tidy graves still taste fire from the rum and realise

the year I left
she died

there's no return.

TEMPERATURE

Piercing breezes
(Sappho Fragment 71)

And it's cold outside. I'm singing
And it's cold outside.
The fan-folds open to pale blue
as a solitary bird flies
to the corner of the parchment

and in my mind
the pages have been turned on
and the dates have gone
angles are forever shifting
and the temperature swings
to this burning hour of frost, loss.

HIROSHIMA

someone will remember us
(Sappho Fragment 147)

The seemingly silent sea warmed
by the unrelenting sun. We stand
wait for a sign that earth will not break.
No rain for weeks dried river, fretting monkeys
and a mackerel-finished sky. Miya-Jima
is in colour today a national holiday.
Cherry blossom begins to confetti the island;
we climb slowly upwards to the Temple.
Time hangs over the edge of snow
still on mountains and the sea far below.
We choose a candle from the box
hope we've interpreted the signs
select one for the family. We pay yen
write your name, light this emblem high
in unfamiliar lands.

HOT TEA

Me … For I'm sure you know how I cherished you
(Sappho Fragment 94)

The oak-scrubbed table is now clear for supper.
We need to home in on the day.
You first, you say. You smile. I hold forth on this and that.

In a dog-rose garden we watch the evening disappear.
And it's your turn. We agree
some things are meant, insights that preserve the sound

of a particular moment, before knowledge, before fear.
You say, *Cheers!* and mugs clink – just enough
to catch the chink of cheap china. Hot Tea.

PHONING TAIPEI

... and what wonderful times we had.
When you walked at my side ...
(Sappho Fragment 94)

And we talked of the stars and how each of us
is stardust. Dust from the same stars we wondered
It's odd, you said, *to think that stars are dead*
for thousands of years before their light shines through.

And like Sappho, you spoke in fragments and left me
to guess. The further out we look into the sky
the further back in time we go. Those were the thoughts
when we had time – time before you left our lives;

but now as I walk to Covent Garden I know you're here.
I'm reliving the gale and how we sheltered to phone Taipei
on a phone card like a final breath about to expire.
Remember the laughter. The expectation. Rain raining down.

WARM DAYS

Beautiful gifts children
(Sappho Fragment 58)

I have this dream a few times;
then I wake.
These are the last warm days
You are here as sunlight through the trees
in clouds that lift the mountains and the hand
that touches faces as we sleep. But you are thinner
than before, more bewildered. You wear
your old grey coat, no doubt to warm your bones.
You stand apart from them (but so much still a part of us)
and there's this whispering though the leaves
The dead can't swim
And the living plunge into clear water.

ERRANDS

and on the ground the purple flower
(Sappho Fragment 105A)

At Goudhurst I stop and buy Green Tea
before entering the churchyard.
Here graves are not guarded by statues.
I leave no money to ward off evil spirits.
I unpick stitches of your last morning;
you leave the boat for that errand, tea half-drunk.
As I walk to your plot an old school-bus stops
at the end of the lane, collects children
for home. Symbols on Taipei's dilapidated buses
had been impossible to decipher
and we ran, laughed, not knowing
how to recognise signs that we needed.

I could walk to your grave blindfolded.
The ground needs to settle in a way you never did.
You found our bus by holding up the paper
to an elderly man who led us forward.
The driver took his fare out of our purse
and we were on our way to buy bean curd.
We rode through shadowed landscapes –
hills rising out of earthquaked lands.
The tofu in the market made our stomachs heave.
Here, stillness, head stones.
Steps on concrete the only winter sound
and I walk alone, carry one small tree.

SPLINTERING THE DARK

And in it cold water makes a clear sound
(Sappho Fragment 2)

Out and beyond the reach of Fridays, the Grand Union Canal
leaves the tail end of yesterday and the Margaret Rose *rests*

while others turn handles on locks, pass through.
Water like a gentle cliché laps through the hours.

No one comes to breathe life into an evening.
Rain splashes sideways across the narrow boat window.

Twilight. A week after the storm
geraniums on the boat bloom and stars splinter the dark.

A young girl walks where holes were dug for poems.
She pauses at the willow where words are buried with roots.

She reads the plaque for her sister whose boat
rocks by the water's edge

and up on the bridge, cars roar past.
These roots with poems will multiply –

earth and leaves will be eaten by worms.
Will sprout up fresh with grass and become the song of thrushes.

HAZY WITH STARS

with roses the whole place is shadowed
(Sappho Fragment 2)

Red roses and ferns in my hands
a cup of Earl Grey on the table
cold against the heat of the night.
I wait for days to turn to autumn.

Sweet peas have lost their mauve
the pink has grown dusty.
Everyone's in bed, the cat sleeps on the grass
a butterfly is white in a night hazy with stars.

TOMORROW

dawn with arms of roses
(Sappho Fragment 58)

I like to think you're out there –
some bar or other waiting for someone
not my business who – but I like to think
you're full of expectation.
At a table for one, you're on a second pint
but ready to slow down when he arrives.
The book can be easily put aside.

And then I see the stairs I'm climbing.
Prepare for bed, block out the picture postcard
Wish you were here.
If you could, would you send that message now
as merged between earth and sky you no longer
talk to us, however hard we try. Always anticipation
for tomorrow. And dawn with arms of roses.

SISTERS

I would rather see her lovely step
And the motion of light on her face
(Sappho Fragment 16)

Your face   her body
her face   your body
                                        once

but now memory   she lies
head cocked to one side at the foot of the churchyard

you thrive on fresh air –
walk the hopfields   carry a hot water bottle
follow
              your dog through woods
to lakes frozen by January ice

but there's no denying she is you

and you now hold her   this weight we need you to carry

it is a burden for you to live up to – we know that

your grief hurricanes you through countrysides
tracks down paths she may have trod   crunch of snow
hard frosts

nothing deters you   you will find your way back –
led by a Labrador who sniffs through bracken

in the winter haze   leaps
   leaps   through trees' shadows
searches   ensures you're following

waits for a ghost round corners   presumes it listens or fades elsewhere or maybe a ghost will leaf through trees leading us

there is this need to touch a ghost and ask do you always follow the same path

how to look at these woods   a close-up neglects the wider view –
an expanse of oaks form a pattern to close the world   keep ghosts apart

ghosts who roam and fly above a tangle of roots and branches or
                                                            do we see each tree   as her
      branches bent in the wind to listen   head raised   the newest shoot

you began your journey twenty-eight years ago as you
                                                                  but to your mother you return as
two

BUT

so we may see
(Sappho Fragment 6)

it’s the silence in the walls;
the language of the bricks
the chimney flue and the muffled cry
with only the odd sigh escaping into night
beyond The Plough over oceans to your early
evening snows (melting the land between us)
that keeps me wanting to know.